Accessible Trails in Chickamauga Park

some hiking, walking and accessible trails for everyone
in the
Chickamauga & Chattanooga National Military Park

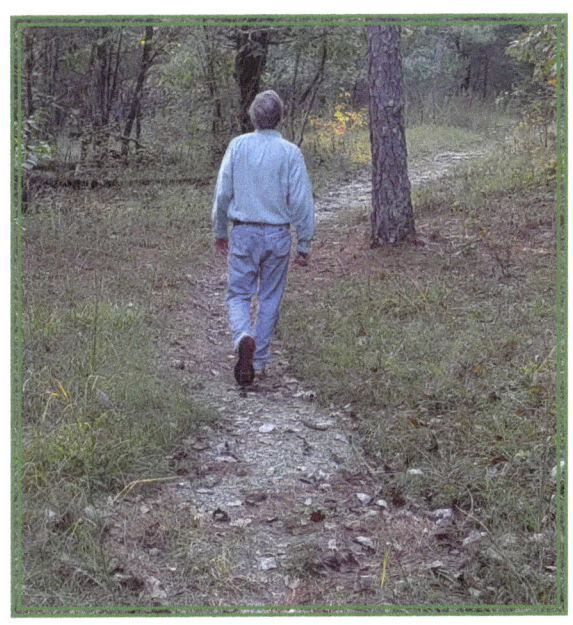

M. Wade Wright

Waldenhouse Publishers, Inc.
Walden, Tennessee

Accessible Trails in Chickamauga Park: *some hiking, walking and accessible trails for everyone in the Chickamauga & Chattanooga National Military Park*

Copyright ©2020 Mary Wade Wright, 1952 All rights reserved. No part of this book may be reproduced in any form or by any electronic or mechanical means including information storage and retrieval systems, without permission in writing from the publisher. The only exception is by a reviewer, who may quote short excerpts in a review.

Published by Waldenhouse Publishers, Inc.
100 Clegg Street, Signal Mountain, Tennessee, USA
888-222-8228   www.waldenhouse.com
Printed in the United States of America
Type and Design by Karen Paul Stone
ISBN: 978-1-947589-36-0

> A summary of fourteen trails in the Chickamauga & Chattanooga National Military Park in southeastern Tennessee and northwest Georgia. Describes access locations and terrain and explains which trails are accessible by wheelchair and which are more rugged.

SPO018000   SPORTS & RECREATION / Hiking
SPO050000   SPORTS & RECREATION / Walking
HEA007000   HEALTH & FITNESS / Exercise / General

TO

Charlie
without whom this could not have been done

CONTENTS

INTRODUCTION	7
TRAIL ONE	9
TRAIL TWO	13
TRAIL THREE	17
TRAIL FOUR	19
TRAIL FIVE	21
TRAIL SIX	23
TRAIL SEVEN	25
TRAIL EIGHT	27
TRAIL NINE	29
TRAIN TEN	31
TRAIL ELEVEN	33
TRAIL TWELVE	35
TRAIL THIRTEEN	37
TRAIL FOURTEEN	39
Project Certificate #1	41
Project Certificate #2	43
Additional Notes	45
Additional Notes	47

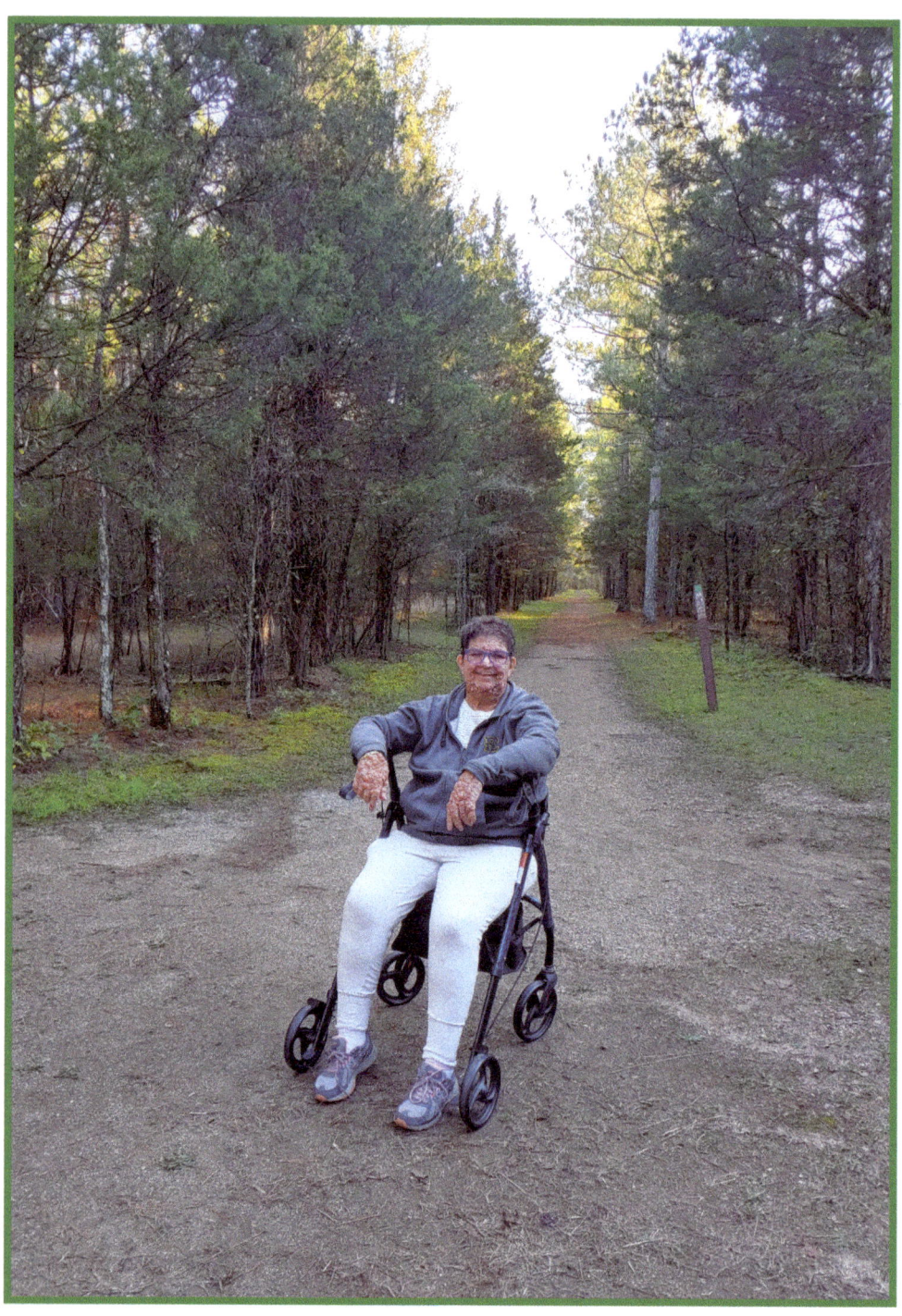

The author's friend Angy Spaulding

INTRODUCTION

The Battle of Chickamauga was one of the bloodiest of the Civil War. Today the Chickamauga & Chattanooga National Military Park is well-kept, and monuments from each state represented are everywhere. As my husband, Charlie, and I have walked through the different paths, we have been amazed at how many new monuments and markers have appeared in just the last year. The first thing I began to notice was that instead of one huge monument, many little white Tennessee markers began appearing everywhere. For a few days, they seemed to be on every trail on which we walked.

The Chickamauga Battlefield trails in this book are marked at the beginning as to what kind of person, animal, or bike can be on the trail. Some are for hikers only, some for walkers and dogs on a leash. Others are accessible also for bicycles or for horses. On some of the horse trails, we have encountered gigantic flies which buzzed past us like a buzzing saw.

I have tried to show some of the trails in this booklet; there is no way I could show every single one. I don't have a pedometer, but have tried to show how long a good hike can take on a trail. I have attempted to show as much as possible (1) the terrain – hilly or flat, (2) if there are places with a lot of tree roots to give some people problems, (3) if the trail is earthen, gravel, sandy, or paved, (4) if it is wide or narrow, and so on. I am trying as much as possible to identify rugged trails that adventurous people and young adults would find rewarding, as well as easy trails that senior citizens would enjoy. Also, if a handicapped person, say in a wheelchair or with a cane, wants to use a trail, I am trying to identify that as well.

Life brings changes, and I would not be surprised to see the Park Service make changes to the descriptions I have provided after this book prints, either making some trails more accessible to wheelchairs, or adding monuments to the trail(s).

8 Accessible Trails in Chickamauga Park

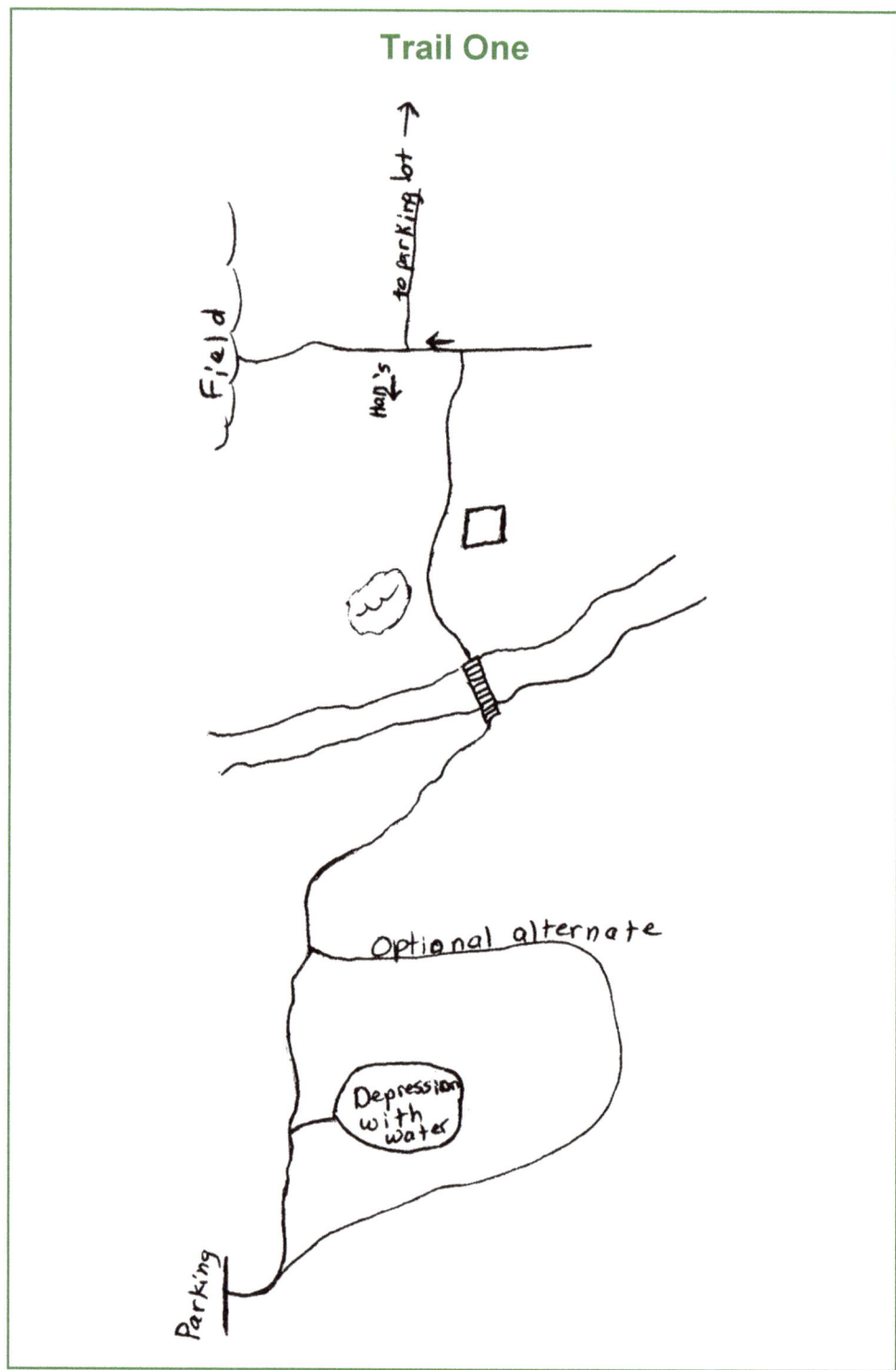

TRAIL ONE Rugged. No wheelchairs.

(1) Both hilly and flat.

(2) Some places in the path have tree roots; others do not, or the forestry people have built walkways to cover.

(3) Pretty much an earthen trail except where forestry additions have been added.

(4) In some places two or three people could be side by side, but in many places it is a single-person trail.

This is a beautiful trail, but is **for people who are sure-footed.** It is very scenic, and goes downhill and up, not just a straight path.

Location: Driving south on LaFayette Road, just past Viniard Alexander Road, take the next left into a double parking place in front of yellow bars blocking any further entrance by vehicle. Get out and walk around the yellow bars, and bear left about eight? feet into the area.

Optional Sideline: After going down the trail about three minutes or so, you can turn right, walk carefully (I wouldn't do this if you have a baby or toddler), and you will soon come to a beautiful depression – a little lake unto itself. Then you have to go back to the trail.

After being on the trail 6 minutes (about 3 minutes if you came back from the sinkhole and started again), you come to an area where the forestry people put down logs, earth, and gravel to help it be more sure footed.

At 7 minutes, you start seeing a creek, or tributary.

At 11 minutes, you have to jump a narrow creek "inlet" (it was dry when we were there.)

At 13 minutes you come to a narrow bridge which crosses the creek.

After crossing the creek and continuing on, you pass a little pond on the left. Across from it on your right is the foundation for a building that has trees and brush growing in it.

The trail comes to a T where you turn left or right. The right turn goes to a wilder section. We turned left. As we continued, we passed a right turn which ends in a parking lot. Just beyond that is a sign pointing left to Hall's House which we also passed.

At 26 minutes we reached a field which is part of the Battlefield, and turned around. At 30 minutes we were at the "T" again and turned right to go back to the bridge.

After crossing the bridge, etc., and going back on the trail, we turned left at a marker for an alternate route around the sinkhole (this is optional; you don't have to do this. You can just follow the first trail back if you want to do so.) This optional trail was a one person at a time trail; then there was a place where they added a two-post bridge affair to walk on and avoid low-lying dirt.

This trail eventually comes back to the starting point like the first trail. You CAN walk down and around the area from this trail, but do be careful. Again, no small children near the sinkhole area. We just kept going on the trail and came back to the starting point of the hike.

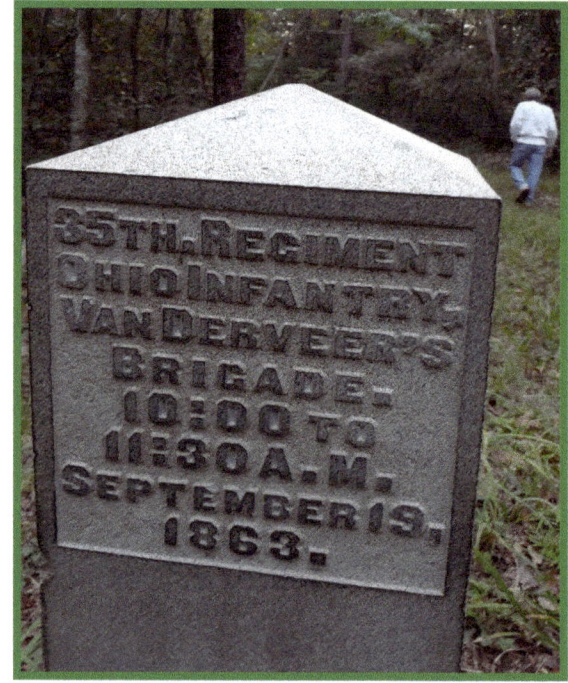

The Battle of Chickamauga was one of the bloodiest of the Civil War. Monuments from each state engaged are placed throughout the National Military Park. Trails pass beside some of these monuments.

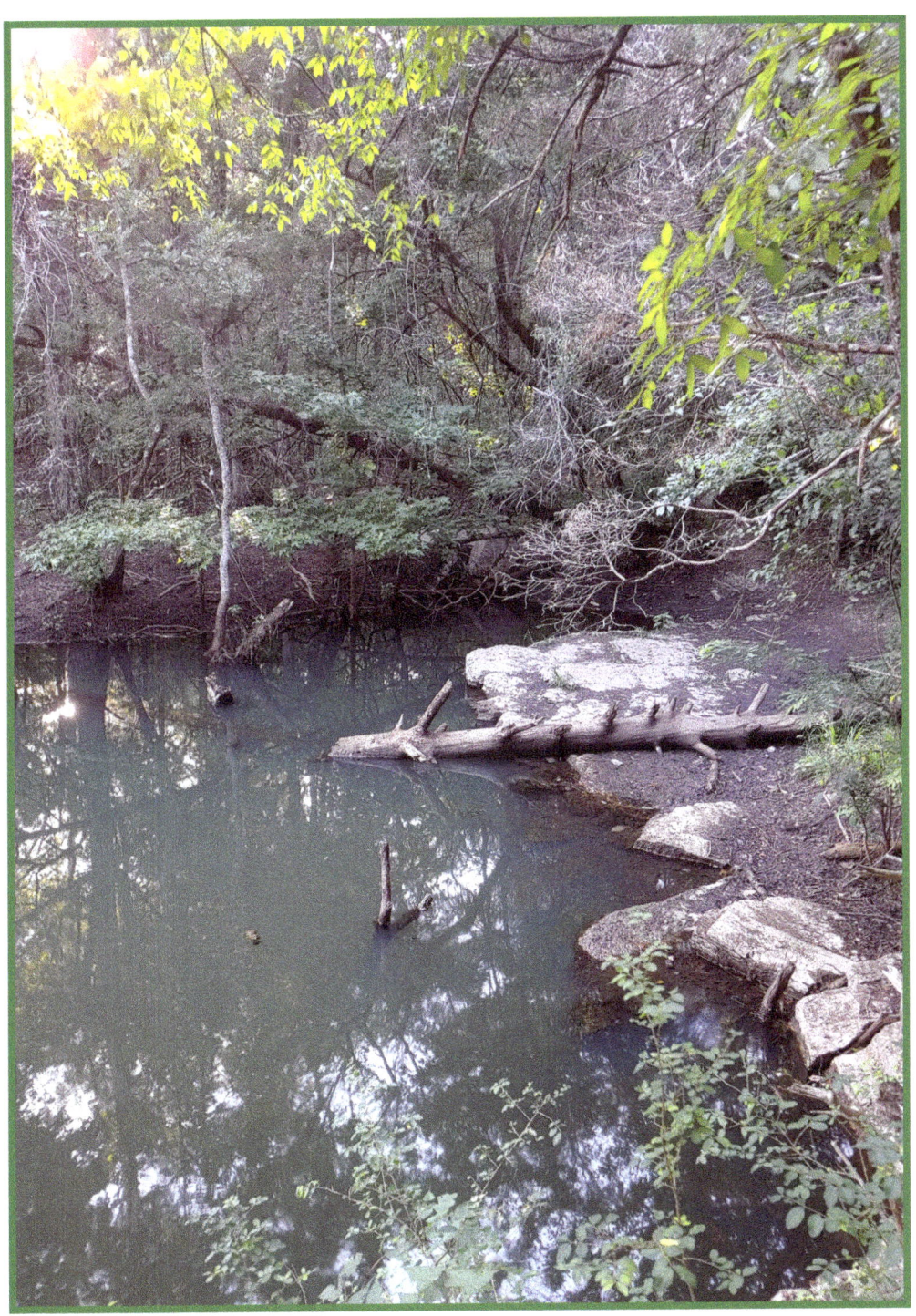
The creek on TRAIL ONE

12 Accessible Trails in Chickamauga Park

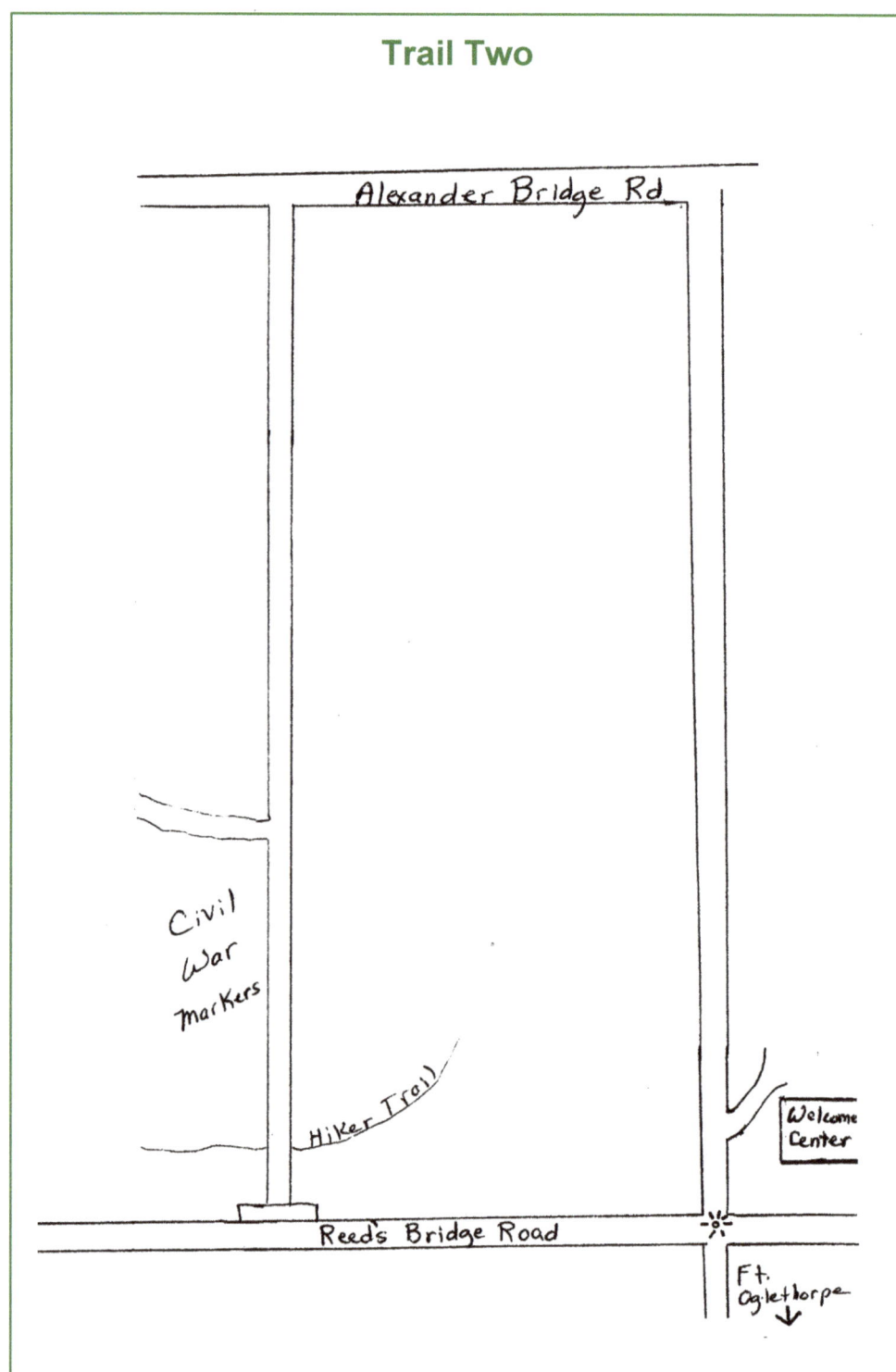

TRAIL TWO. Nice and wide. Not many tree roots. No horses or bikes. You can probably bring your dog on a leash if you also have a bag for collecting and disposing of waste.

(1) This is basically flat. If you're in a wheelchair there may be an upward or downward grade, but I didn't notice one except near the entrances.

(2) This path is an old road, and is level. Not many tree roots at all.

(3) This is not paved, but is nice and leveled out, sometimes pine needles covering, sometimes small gravel. Also earth.

(4) This is a nice, wide trail! Four people could easily walk side by side.

This trail is user friendly, and basically straight.

Location: If you are headed south from Ft. Oglethorpe, turn left at the red light before the Park's Welcome Center onto Reeds Bridge Road. If you are coming up from Chickamauga, pass the Welcome Center and turn right at the red light onto Reeds Bridge Road. Where you see the statue of a man with a rammer for a cannon across from Forrest Road's dead end (this is a Tennessee monument), park in the parking spaces that are there, lock your vehicle, and go up to the entrance to the forest. **Wheelchair people may elect to use the south entrance off of Alexander Bridge Road** east of the sign at the road that says "Helm monument 200 ft; Colquite Monument 335 ft." This is several feet eastward and has a more gradual uphill slope, although longer.

One minute in from Reeds Bridge Road, there is an optional ↔ hiker trail. We did not take it, and stayed straight on the main trail. This hiker trail is later described in Trail Thirteen.

Mainly on the left, but also on the right, there are occasional Civil War markers and explanations. At one place there are also two cannons.

About halfway down, another road goes off of the main path, and if you have the time and energy, it is worth your walk. It passes more Civil War markers and is another ten minutes or so until it dead ends into a road that goes two ways; we turned around at Helm marker and came back up. If you have all day, you can try the road. We timed the walk all the way to Alexander Bridge Road first, and took this turnoff coming back.

It took us thirteen minutes from the start off of Reeds Bridge Road to the south end near Alexander Bridge Road, and another minute for me to walk down to the signs "Helm monument 200 feet; Colquitt Monument 335 feet." Walking back to Reeds Bridge Road would be another thirteen minutes unless you want to take the road off of the main path described above and add some more minutes. Also, at Alexander Bridge Road across the street, there are more markers and another road.

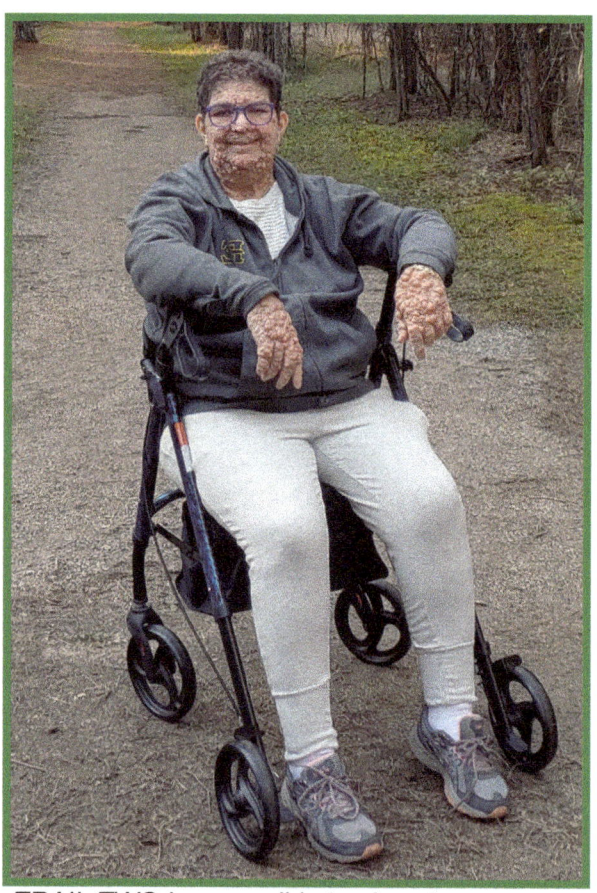

TRAIL TWO is accessible to almost anyone, as Angy Spaulding demonstrates.

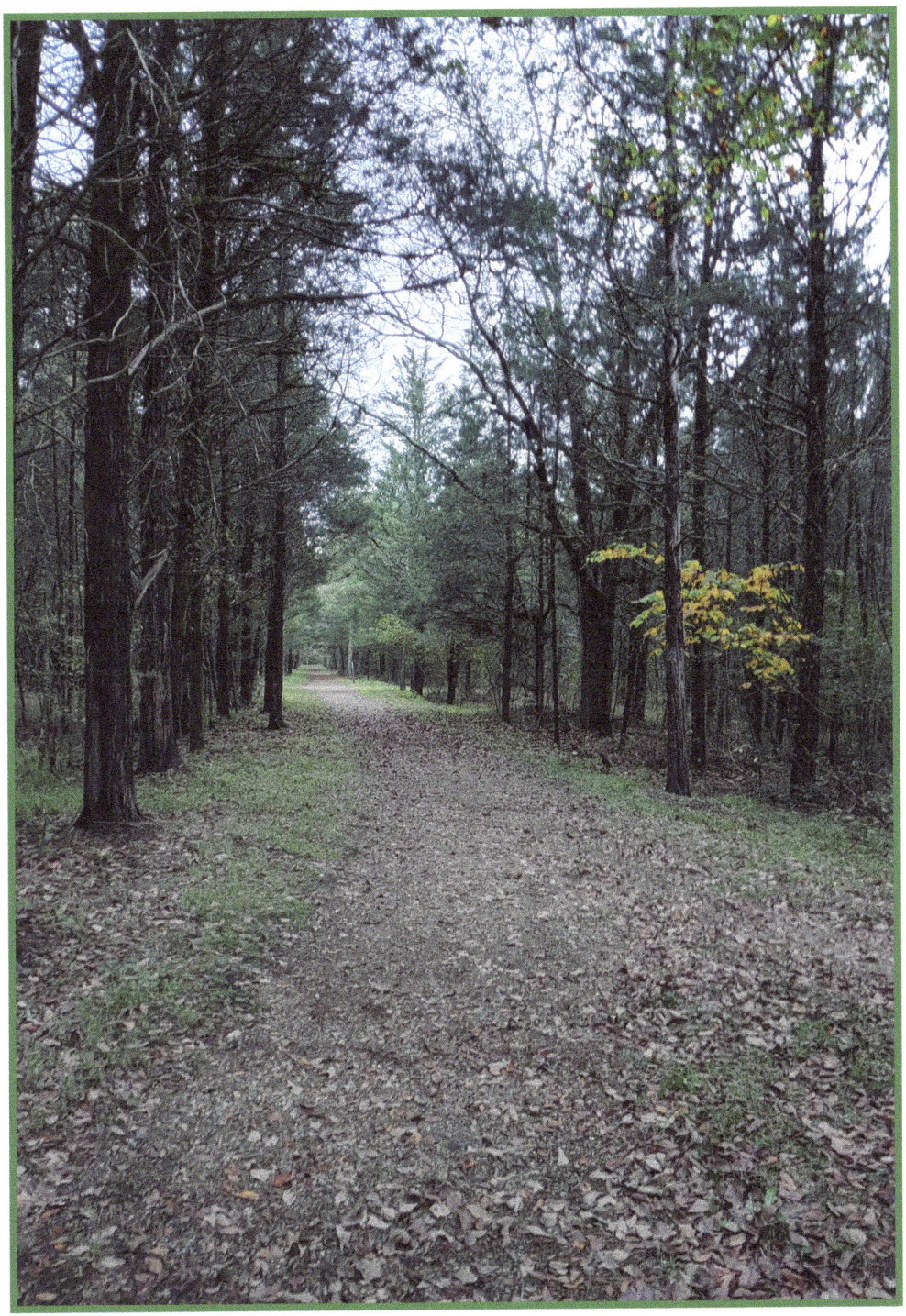
TRAIL TWO Is nice, wide and fairly level

Trail Three

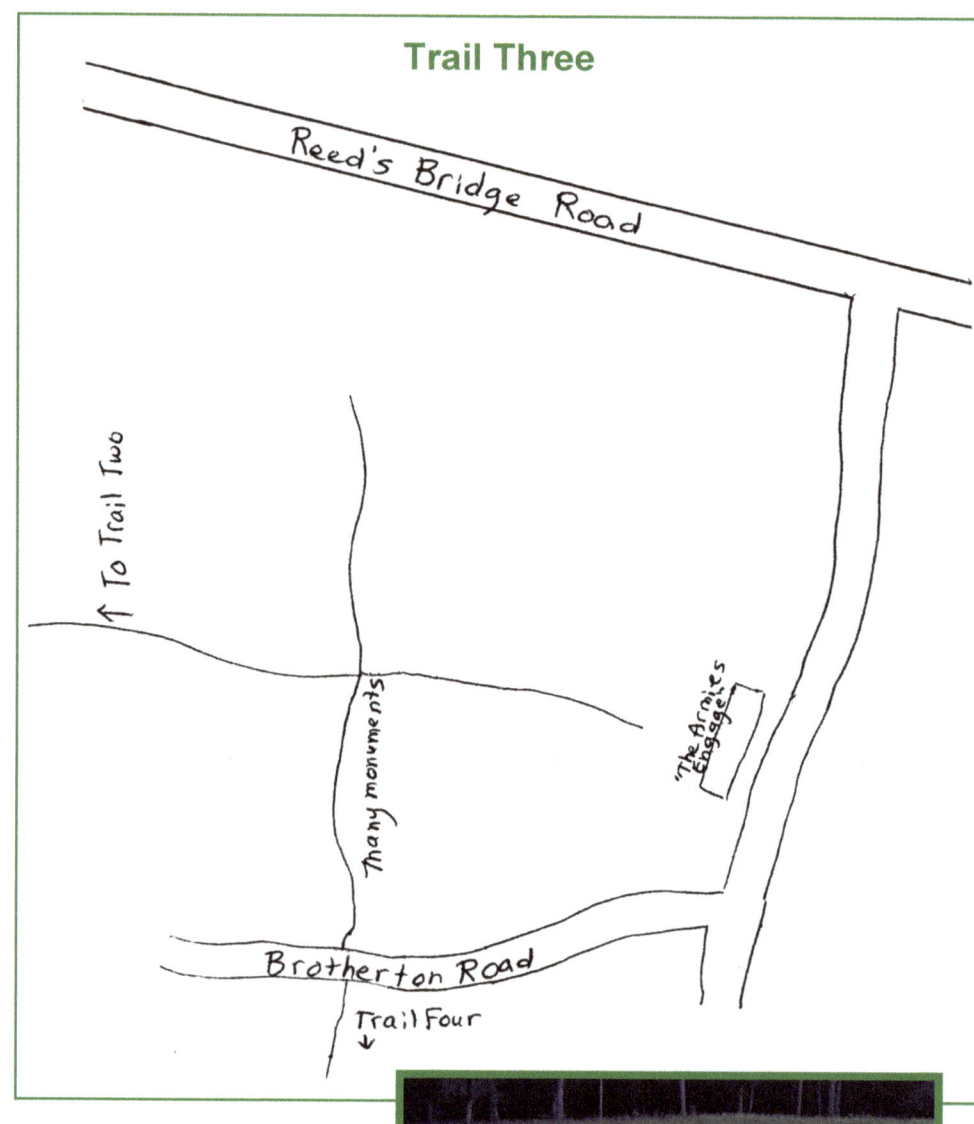

This sign at the starting point for TRAIL THREE points to where Jay's Mill used to be located.

TRAIL THREE. No horse or bike. Dog on leash is OK. Trail Three starts on Jay's Mill Road.

(1)(2) This trail goes up hill and down. Sorry, no wheelchairs; there are some very bad places for wheelchairs. People with canes will need to watch their step, as in some places there are many stones and in other places a lot of tree roots. Ironically, there are also places where the path is nice and broad, with not a lot of stones or tree roots.

(3) Obviously this is not paved.

(4) This is a former road, and in most places it is nice and wide for walking, although there are a few places where gullies have appeared and you have to walk very carefully. Even younger adults have to be careful here.

Location: From Reeds Bridge Road, turn onto Jay's Mill road. TRAIL THREE starts from a flagstone landing where there is a description of the fighting entitled, "The Armies Engage." After about 17 minutes, at the top of a hill, there is an intersection. If you go straight, after 38 more minutes you will reach the Gen. Helm marker mentioned at the turnaround on TRAIL TWO.

If you turn right at this intersection, it will eventually go to Reeds Bridge Road.

If you turn left at this intersection, it will eventually go to Brotherton Road. One of the monuments on this trail is Burnham's Battery H. 5th U.S. Artillery. If you have plenty of time for walking and it is not about to get dark, this left turn has some other monuments and is a nice, long walk.

When you reach the paved road (Brotherton), turn left and you will walk down Brotherton to where it intersects Reeds Bridge Road. I was able to see my car as we neared Reeds Bridge Road, as it was parked near the flagstone landing with the description called "The Armies Engage."

Another note: If it is early in the day and you want to walk some more, cross Brotherton instead of turning left, and the trail with the monuments continues.

Trail Four

↑ Trail Three ↓

Brotherton Road

Trail Four ↓

Bragg's Hdqtrs

Jay's Mill Road

Alexander's Bridge Road

TRAIL FOUR Horses yes, bikes no. Dog on leash OK.

Location: TRAIL FOUR starts at Bragg's Headquarters on Brotherton Road, across from where the TRAIL THREE intersection ends on Brotherton Road.

(1)(2) This trail goes up hill and down gradually like the "left turn at intersection" trail on TRAIL THREE, and is a nice walk.

Wheelchairs OK around Bragg's Headquarters, but not after that. People with canes will need to watch their step.

Occasional roots in path. In one place, about halfway down, there is a wet weather creek, but in dry weather only stones to cross.

(3) This is not paved. There is gravel in some places, just dirt in others.

(4) This is another former road, and in several places people can walk comfortably three abreast.

Walking to where the trail dead-ended on Alexander Bridge Road and back to the beginning took a total of 47 minutes.

There is a memorial sign on this trail to Fowler's Alabama Battery who at one point fought alongside an Arkansas regiment. There are a couple of other memorials also, one of which you have to leave the path and go in about thirty feet to see.

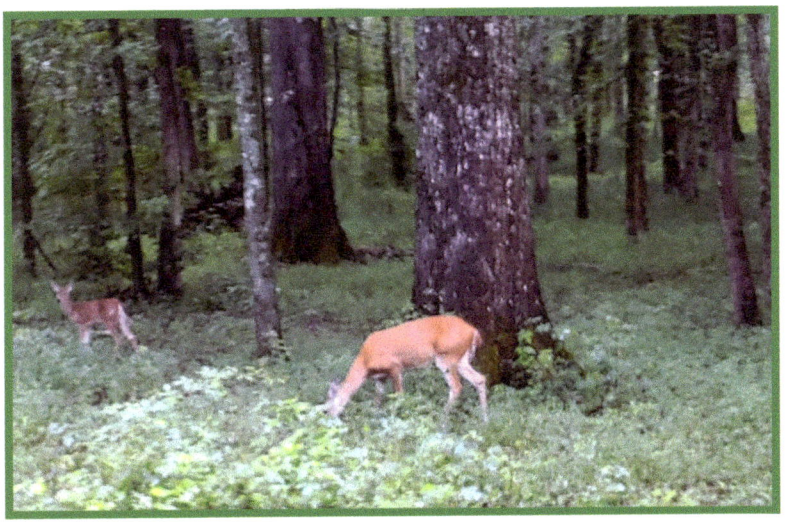

Seeing deer and other wildlife is a bonus for visitors.

Trail Five

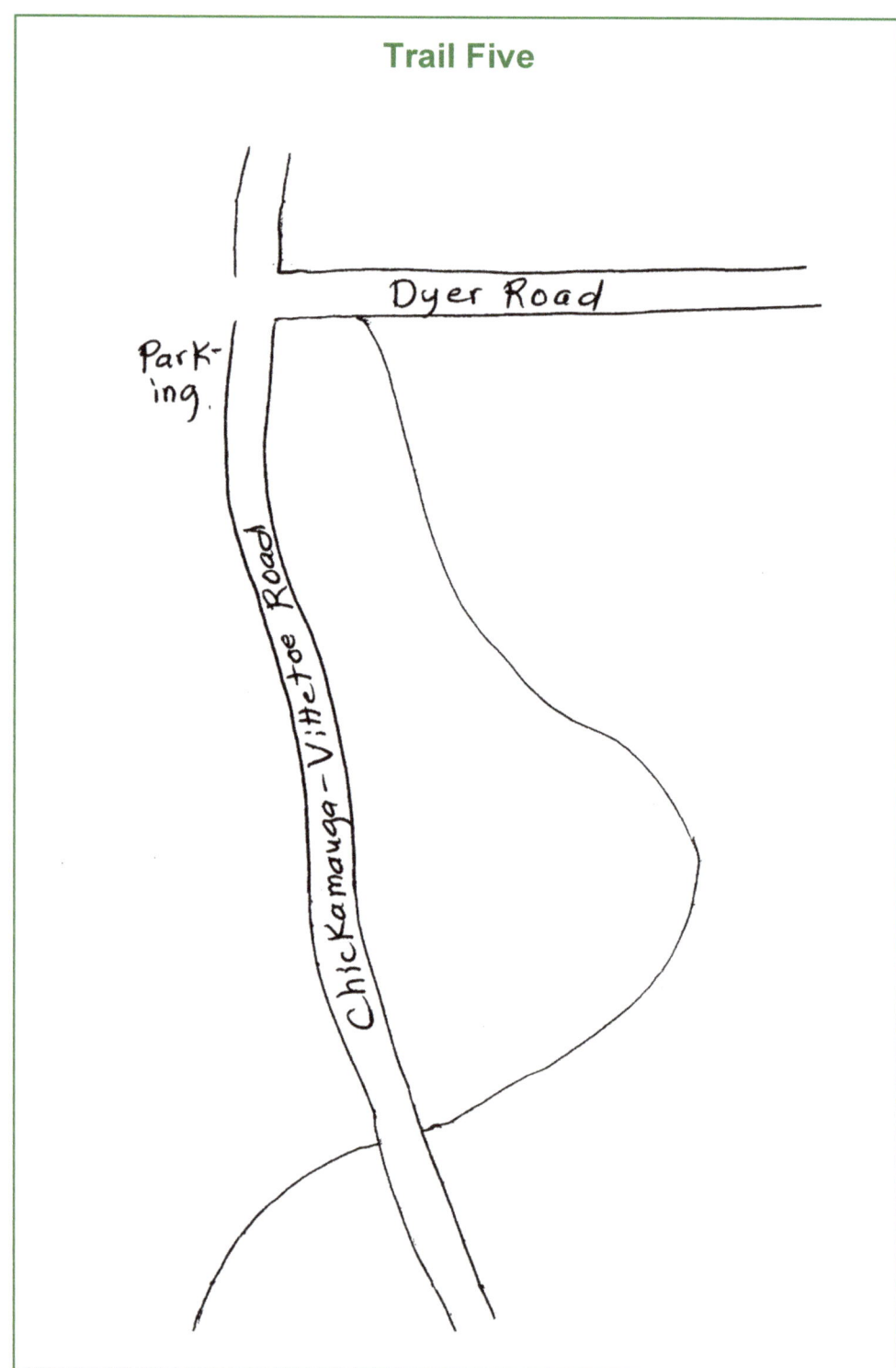

TRAIL FIVE Horses yes, bikes no. Dog on leash OK. No wheelchairs, but people in wheelchairs can drive or be dropped off one quarter of a mile down Chickamauga-Vittetoe Road to see monuments. Brig. Gen. William Lytle's marker, though, is on the crest of the hill.

Location: Trail Five starts from Dyer Road. From the Visitors' Center, head South on LaFayette Road through the Battlefield and turn right on Dyer Road. At the stop sign, go straight. Cross Chickamauga-Vittetoe and park in the parking area. From here walk back up the hill 1/10 mile from the parking area to the starting point.

(1)(2) This trail goes up the hill where Brig. Gen. William Lytle's marker and some other markers are, then back down to Chickamauga-Vittetoe Road at the "one quarter of a mile" mentioned above. The monuments mentioned above are across Chickamauga-Vittetoe Road, and then a path which is another converted old road and wider in some places than in others. People with canes will need to watch their step. Occasional roots in path.

(3) This is not paved. There is gravel in some places, just dirt in others.

(4) This is another former road, and in several places people can walk comfortably three abreast.

The starting point leaves Dyer Road and goes up an earthen and tree pole walkway, then across a field on a cow path affair. It then goes up a hill to where Brig. Gen. William Lytle's marker is near the military crest, killed 9/20/1863. The trail then goes down through a forest area and crosses Chickamauga-Vittetoe Road, where the markers are on the other side. From there on, the path goes through the woods

There is a memorial sign on this trail to Fowler's Alabama Battery.

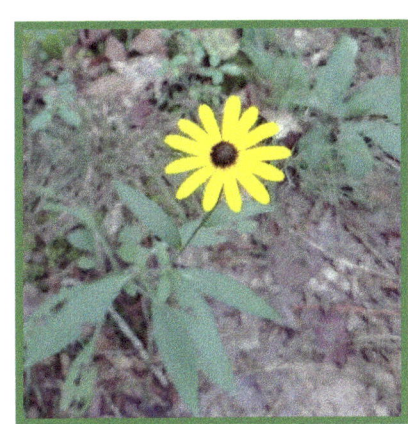

Though once a battleground, the Park and trails are peaceful now.

Trail Six

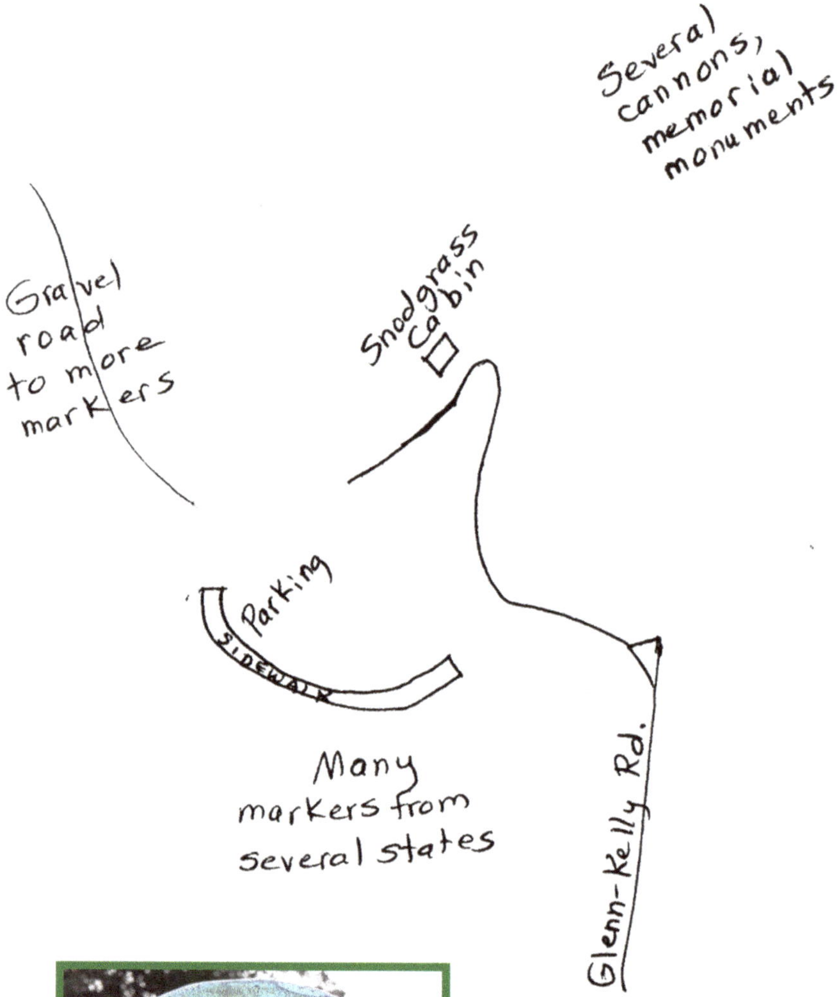

Several cannons, memorial monuments

Gravel road to more markers

Snodgrass Cabin

Parking
SIDEWALK

Many markers from several states

Glenn-Kelly Rd.

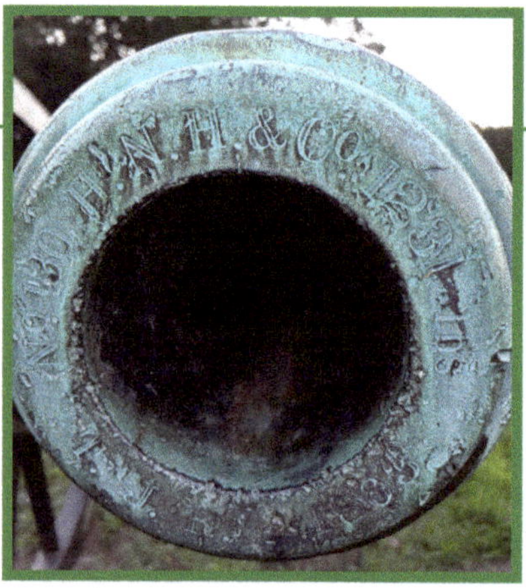

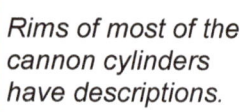

Rims of most of the cannon cylinders have descriptions.

TRAIL SIX Dog on leash OK.

Location: From the Visitors' Center, head South on LaFayette Road through the Battlefield and turn right onto Dyer Road; if you are going north on LaFayette Road from Chickamauga, turn left. Then turn right on Glenn-Kelly Road and you will be headed north. Keep driving until you see a triangular turn on the left hand side, and turn left onto it. The road will go straight, then turn right and wind around to the reconstructed copy of the Snodgrass Cabin.

This served as a Union field hospital during the fighting. The road passes by the cabin and goes to the top of the hill which looks down on three sides. Here there is parking, a sidewalk, and a handicapped parking place. Several markers from several states dot the area.

People in wheelchairs have access to the sidewalk, while those on canes can hike up the grounds to the markers.

To the west, the hill goes on up to more markers, but the road is gravel and there is no sidewalk. I would say hikers only on this hill. On the upper hill from the gravel road the Headquarters Corp was, Major General Gordon Granger.

On the other side of Snodgrass cabin is the field where several Union signs, memorial monuments, and cannons of different sizes are. **No sidewalks, but people with canes and light people in wheelchairs might be able to carefully make their way on a dry day.**

One interesting note is that the edges of most of the cannon cylinders contain descriptions like "J.HVF No. 676 PIC° 1863 316 lbs." They were fascinating, but I couldn't read all of the print on most of them. Each cylinder was different.

Trail Seven

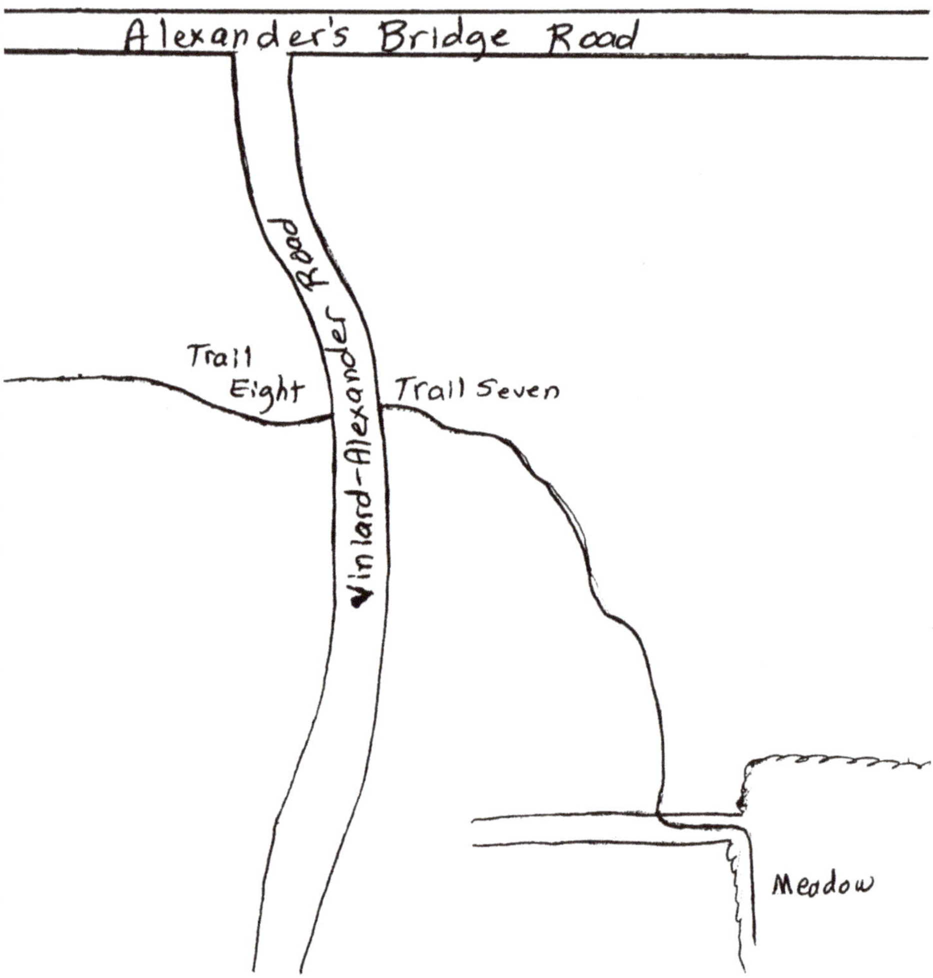

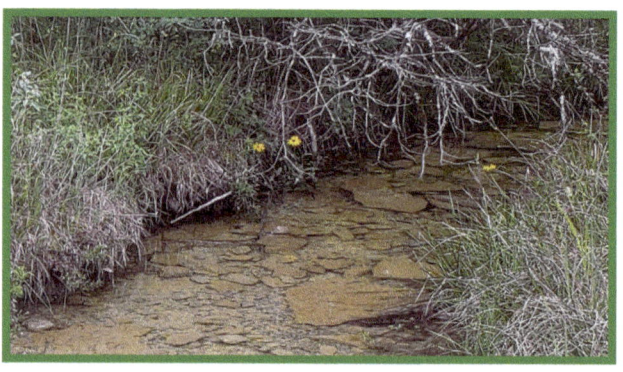

One of several little creeks along the trails

TRAIL SEVEN Hikers only. No animals.

This is a fun hiking trail, somewhat rugged, and crosses two small gullies which are wet-weather creeks. The third is a baby creek.

Location: From Alexander's Bridge Road, turn onto Viniard-Alexander Road. Parking for this is the second dirt-gravel pull-off on the left. For TRAIL SEVEN, turn left. Across the road is TRAIL EIGHT, which is plainly marked for hikers only.

From the road, this trail goes down and continues in a descending manner. If you had looked to the left about a minute before pulling off to park, you would have seen Chickamauga Creek, which then bends so that you don't see it from the trail and would have to go to the left and down to see it.

This is a small trail, so I would stay on the trail. There had been quite a bit of rain before I was on it, so we passed three wet-weather creeks in which the Park people had strategically placed stones on which you can step when it has rained. As stated above, I think one of these always has water in it; the other two are probably dry when it has not rained.

This trail continues to gradually descend, and eventually comes to an old road before emptying onto a meadow owned by the Park Service. If you walk far enough down the meadow by the edge of the woods, you will see a trail with a marker going into the woods, but it was getting to be sunset and we turned back.

POISON IVY WARNING: As we walked on the edge of the meadow near the woods where the Park Service people had cut the grass, I saw baby Poison Ivy plants and steered clear. That was another reason I also didn't leave the trail to go look for the creek in the woods before reaching the meadow; I didn't want to happen upon any Poison Ivy plants in the woods.

If you stay on the path, it is a very pleasant walk. It took us 50 minutes to walk down to the meadow and back to the car; not bad. I would say to probably count on an hour.

I did not see any monuments on this trail.

26 *Accessible Trails in Chickamauga Park*

Trail Eight

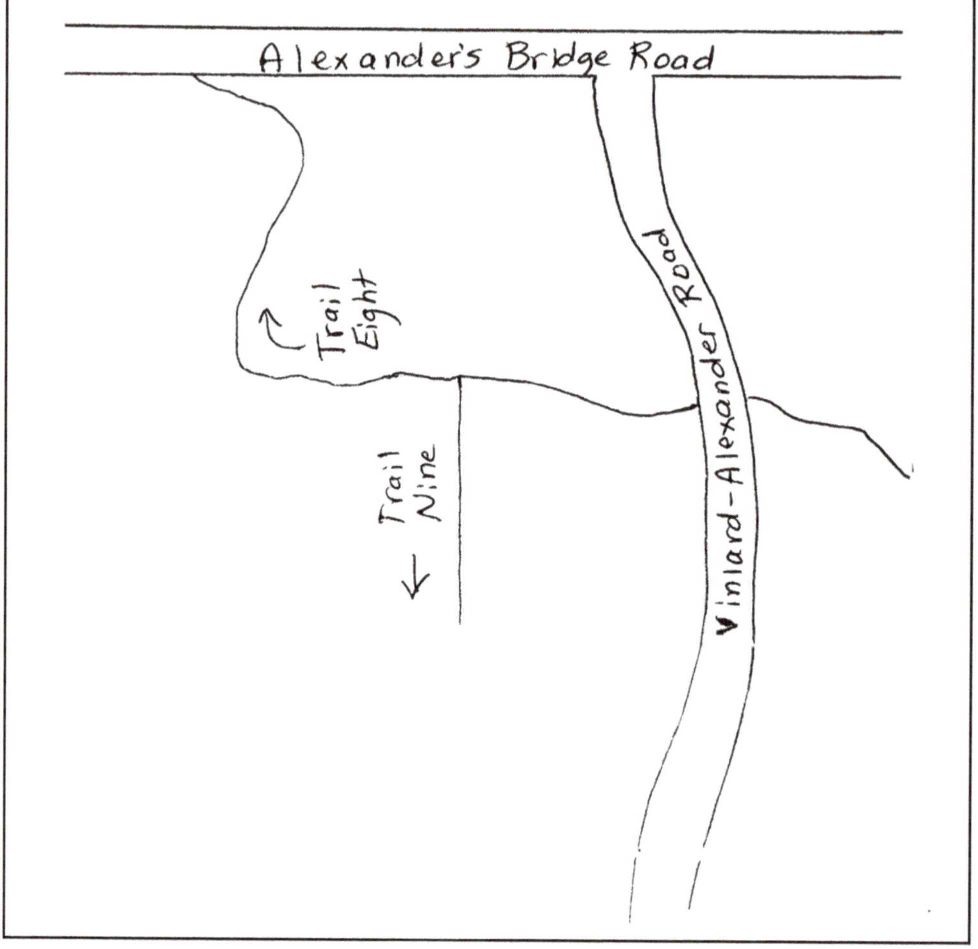

(Hand-drawn map showing Alexander's Bridge Road running horizontally, Viniard-Alexander Road curving down from it, Trail Eight branching off, and Trail Nine extending downward.)

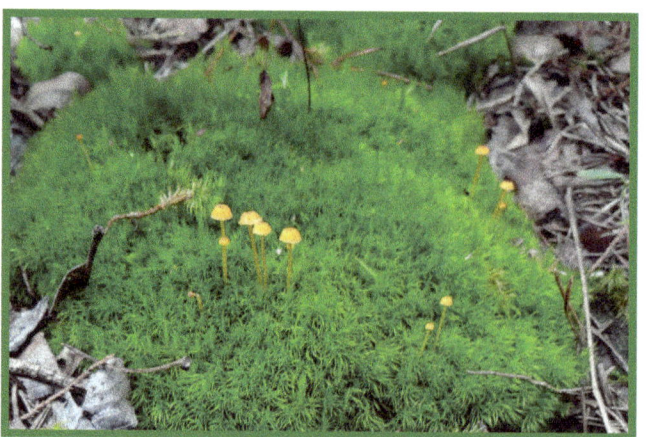

Life in many forms can be seen along the trails.

TRAIL EIGHT Hikers only. No horses or bikes.

This trail is a bit wider than TRAIL SEVEN, and at one point there is a four-way intersection.

For TRAIL EIGHT, we went straight.

Location: Again, for the starting point, from Alexander's Bridge Road, turn onto Viniard-Alexander Road. Parking for this is the second dirt-gravel pull-off on the left.

For TRAIL EIGHT, cross Viniard-Alexander Road to the marker which indicates hikers only.

From Alexander's Bridge Road, take the trail uphill to a bit of a clearing. Where the paths intersect, for TRAIL EIGHT we went straight and into the woods.

In some places the trail is one person only, while in other places two people could probably walk side by side. I did not see any poison ivy, and it was very pleasant. Part of the way through the woods is a sign pointing left with the words, "To Jay's Mill 1 ½ M, Alexander's House 5/8 mi."

We kept on walking until the Trail emptied out onto Alexander's Bridge Road and walked down it and back down Viniard-Alexander Road to the car, although you can go back through the woods if you would rather do so. From the start of the Trail to Alexander's Bridge Road was 30 minutes; walking back to the car by the road was another 25 minutes.

There were no monuments or other markers besides the hikers only sign or the sign "To Jay's Mill…"

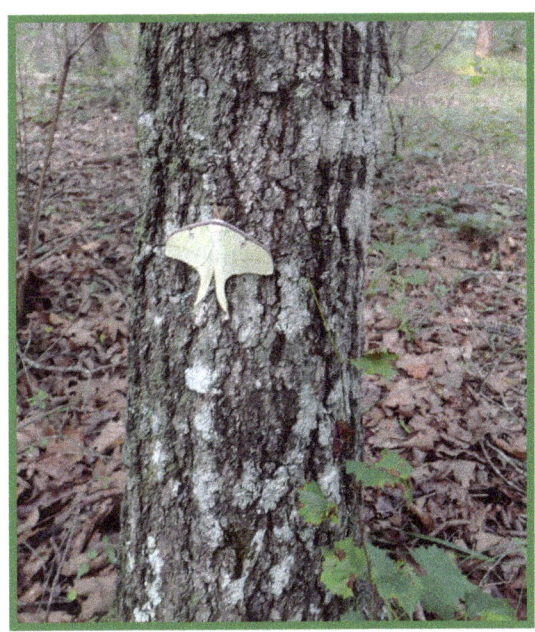

Trail Nine

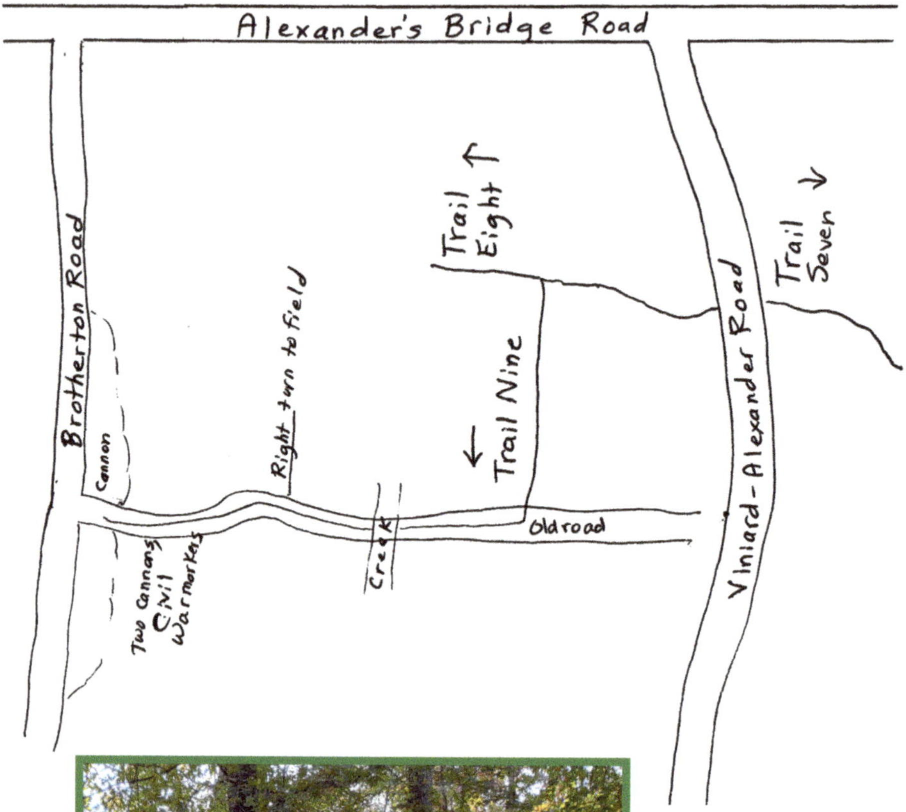

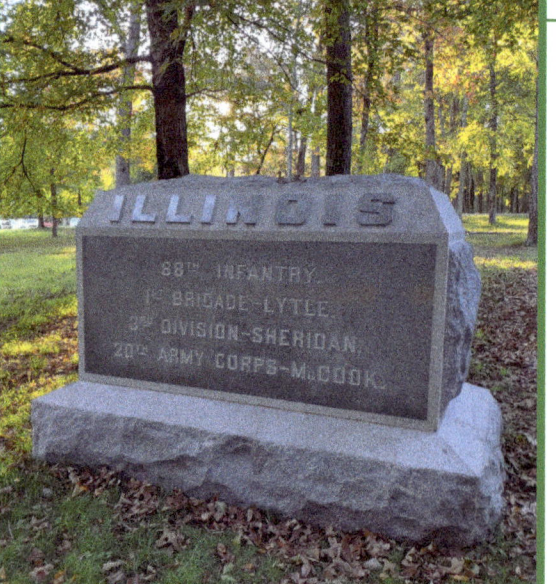

This is one of two monuments to the 88th Infantry Division of Illinois and is located near the activities field on Glen-Kelly Road. More than 50 Infantry Divisions from Illinois fought at Chickamauga.

TRAIL NINE Two entries to this trail. The first one is hikers only. The second one is more accessible to people with canes and wheelchairs.

(1) The first entry begins at Alexander's Bridge Road in the same place as TRAILS SEVEN and EIGHT. For this one, when you get on the same trail as TRAIL EIGHT and get to the clearing where it is rocky and has pretty much just young cedar trees, turn LEFT at the crossroad.

This will go into the woods and eventually dead-end into an old road which is also evidently a path for people with horses. At this dead-end, turn RIGHT onto the old road and follow it. You will go to the right where a small creek flows and pass through it on the rocks, then continue on the path.

When you get to a place where there is a right turn, CONTINUE STRAIGHT onto a small trail. (The right turn is nice, but winds up in a nondescript field.) You will start seeing Civil War markers on this straight path, mainly Confederate. Cheatham's Division – Polk's Corps, Smith's Brigade in Cheatham's Division (Brig. Gen. Preston Smith), etc. There are several along the way. When you see the two cannons, you are not far from the Brotherton Road end of this trail. It continues on the other end of Brotherton Road, but we did not take it.

(2) The second entry begins at the grassy area, one lone cannon, and the CSA Smith's Mississippi Battery… small sign off of Brotherton Road. **People with wheelchairs will need help but can wheel around in dry weather to the cannon. At the entrance to the forest, the hiker trail says no bikes or horses, but people can walk their dogs here. People with canes will have to be careful, but if they are healthy, can walk back in the woods on the trail down to the two cannons. I wouldn't recommend a wheelchair in the woods**.

Personal note: I really wouldn't recommend a horse in the woods; in the very rocky area, I saw horseshoe prints in the dirt, but it would be easy for a horse to lose their footing and injure a foot or leg at some places on this road. I think the "No horses" sign was right.

Trail Ten

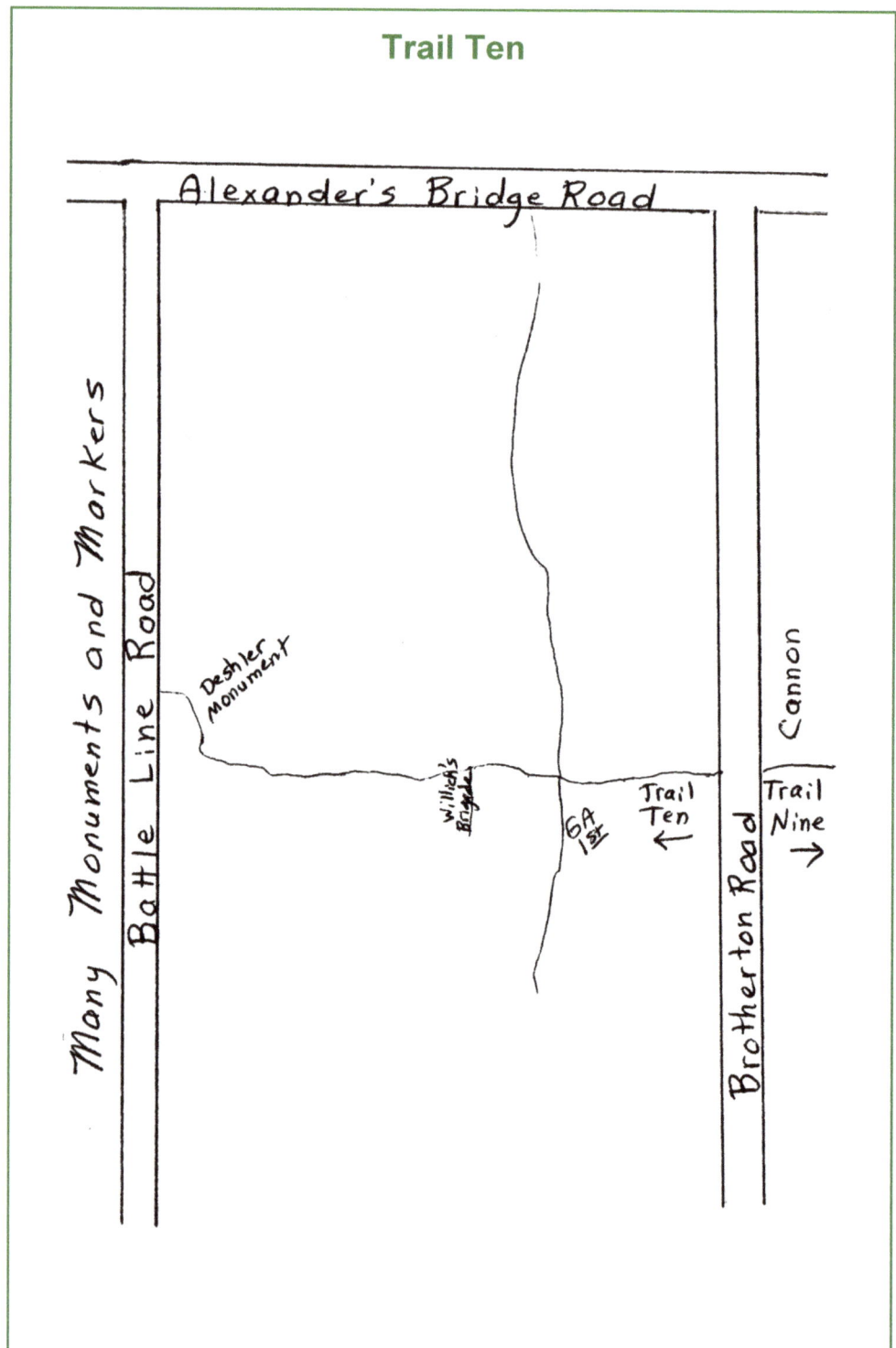

TRAIL TEN   Hikers and people with dogs only. No horses or bicycles.

This trail has some roots and gullies, so no wheelchairs. People with canes will not walk the whole trail, but might walk just a bit.

TRAIL TEN begins across Brotherton Road from TRAIL NINE, and ends on Battle Line Road about 22 minutes later.

Five minutes in, there is a right turn which we did not take, which can take you to Alexander Bridge Road. Across from the right turn is a sign about Cleburn's Division – Hill's Corps (CSA.) If you turn left here and go about 83 paces, you will come to a large CSA marker, Georgia 1st Confederate, 2nd Battalion Infantry. More markers are farther down this "left turn trail" if you are interested.

Back at the main trail, at the Cleburn's Division sign, continue on the main trail. A few minutes farther down on the left is a sign about Willich's Brigade, Johnson's Division (USA.)

Near the end of the trail is the Deshler's Brigade, Cleburne's Division sign, and not far from this sign is the cannonball monument to Brig. General Deshler (CSA) who was shot and killed.

NOTE: Historians as well as people with wheelchairs and canes will greatly enjoy Battle Line Road, where TRAIL TEN ends, with its endless monuments and markers. Cars crawl through this road so people can enjoy the historical markers, comments, and stories on Battle Line Road.

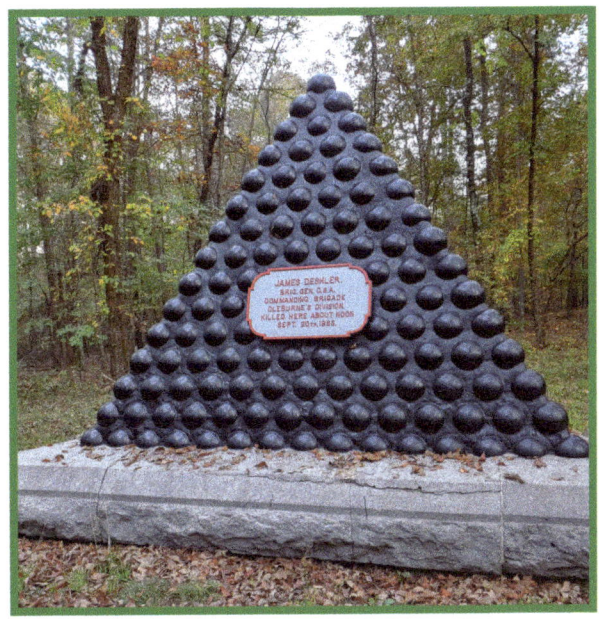

Monument to Brig. General Deshler (CSA)

Trail Eleven

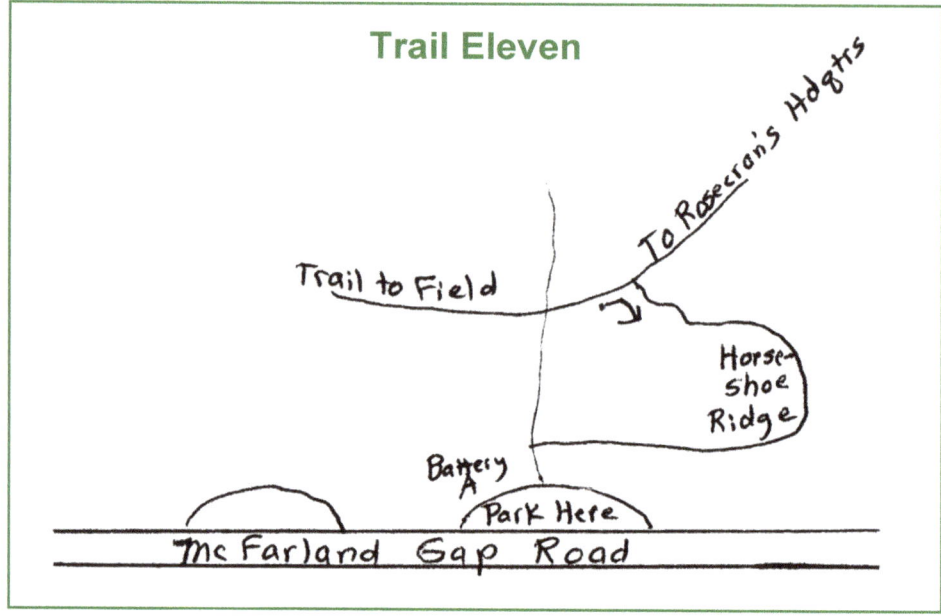

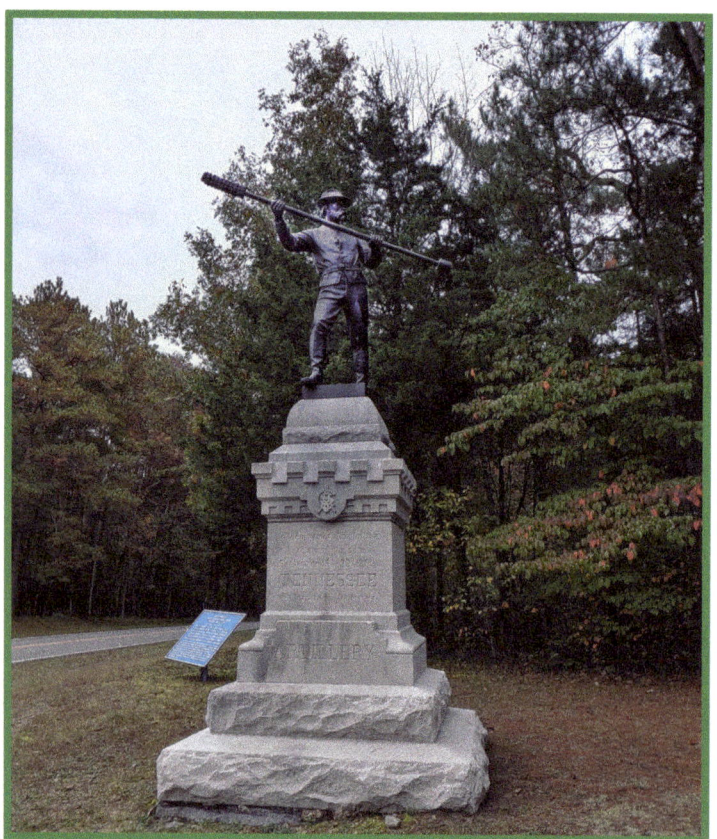

The Tennessee Artillery monument is at Reed's Bridge Road parking area for Trail Two,

TRAIL ELEVEN Hikers, bikes, and people with a dog on a leash. No horses.
This is a narrow trail going south and up a steep hill. No wheelchairs; I don't recommend canes either.

Location: McFarland Gap Road is north of the Visitor Center. Going north, turn left on McFarland Gap Road; if you are coming south from Ft. Oglethorpe, turn right on McFarland Gap Road. When you get on McFarland and pass the field on your left, look for the second left turn with parking spaces.

TRAIL ELEVEN goes south into the woods. When you finally top the hill, to the left is Battery A, First Ohio Light Artillery. A trail goes down the hill past this and toward the field; we did not take it. We came back and turned left going down the trail. Horses are allowed here, and it is wider than it was first coming up the hill.

Further down the trail, we did take a left turn and followed it down a narrow trail like a cattle trail. About five minutes later it opened onto a field, and when you look to the right, you can see Snodgrass Hill, maybe 1/8 of a mile away.

We came back to the original trail, crossed it, and went straight. (If you were coming south and hadn't turned left like we did, it would be a right turn.) If you continue on this trail, it will connect over at Rosecran's headquarters, but we didn't go over there. Instead, after a few minutes we turned right and went up Horseshoe Ridge. Going up at this point is steep. **Hikers only!** No horses. And take your time. After five minutes we were near the top of the ridge; after another five minutes, we reached the very top.

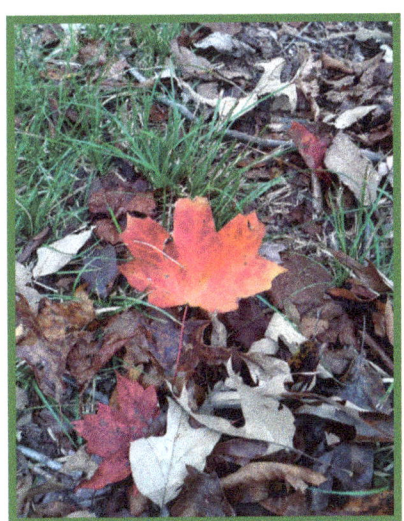

Seven minutes later, we had completed the horseshoe and were back down at the intersection turning left to go back to the start of this hike; after another couple of minutes, we were back at the start.

34 Accessible Trails in Chickamauga Park

Trail Twelve

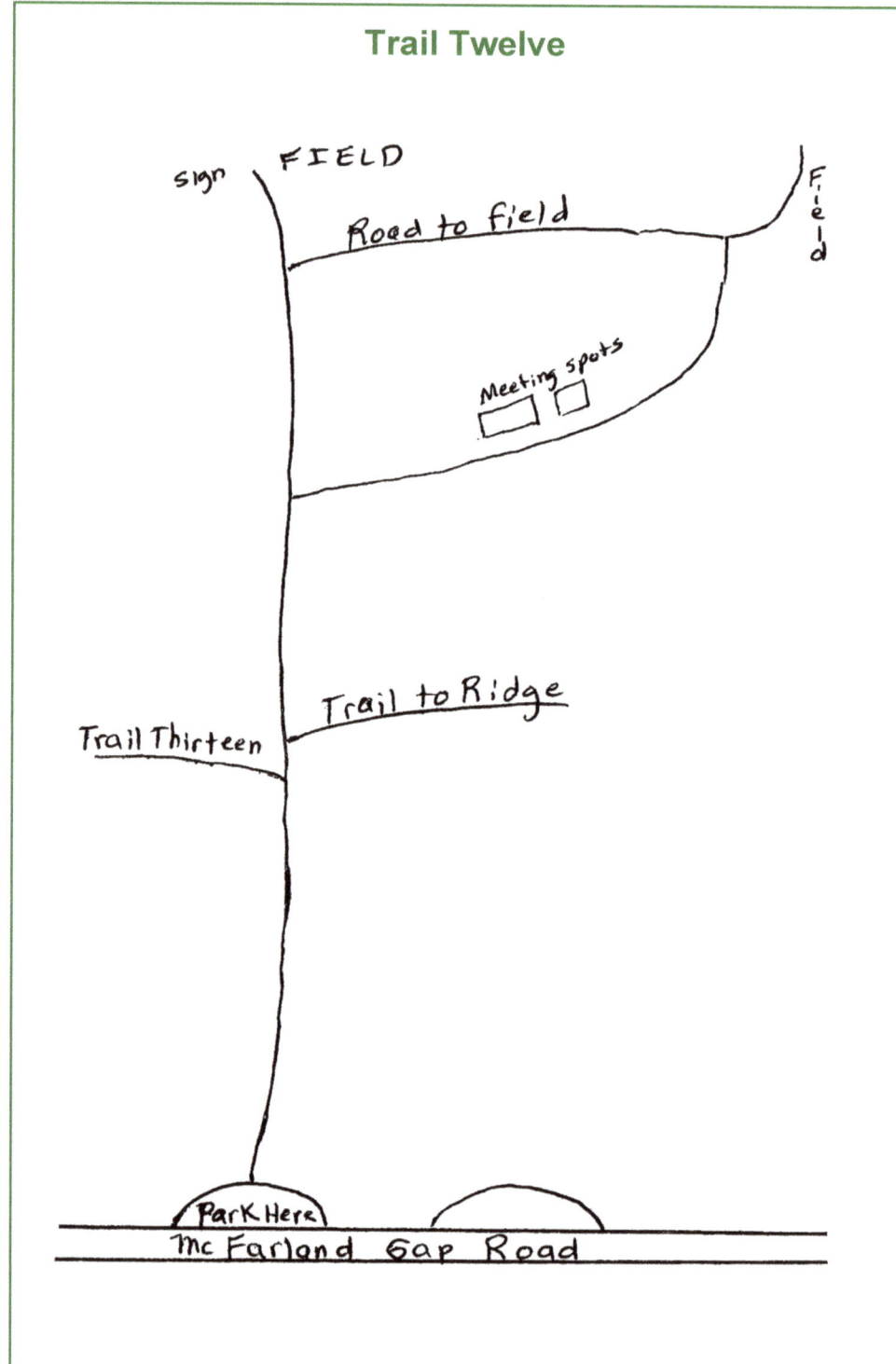

TRAIL TWELVE Wheelchair people can maneuver carefully with assistance. There is a gravel entrance, then asphalt, but it is a service road and has occasional ruts. It isn't smooth, but is serviceable. And TRAIL TWELVE stays level – no big hills.

Location: On McFarland Gap Road, the entrance to this is the first left, before TRAIL ELEVEN.

Being a service road, there are no markers from the Civil War until you get to the entrance to the field on the other end. It is a nice walk, though, and we saw several people as well as people on bicycles.

About six minutes in, there is a trail to the left for hikers or horses – no bikes or cars. This is described later as TRAIL THIRTEEN.

Just after it, to the right, is a trail that leads to Horseshoe Ridge, like on TRAIL ELEVEN. This is also a horse trail. We stayed on the main trail.

Ten minutes in was a right turn which we took later, but we followed the service road first to its end where the field begins. At the borderline between the forest and the field is a barrier to keep non-service cars out and a sign "Withdrawal of the Union Left, Sept. 20, 1863, 5:30 p.m.", with a description of what happened.

(Shortly before the borderline and the barrier sign was a road turning to the right which we later discovered goes to the field under Snodgrass Hill.)

We then walked back to the right turn mentioned earlier and walked on it. The path went through the forest, and we saw a couple of spots to the left which looked like they might be used for open meetings – maybe discussing Civil War reenactments?

The path eventually ended on the road mentioned inside the parentheses above. We turned right and came upon the field below Snodgrass Hill. We followed this road for quite a few minutes to its end at the paved road going to Snodgrass Hill. It and another gravel/dirt road across the street were both marked "Service Road—Do Not Enter." It made for a nice walk, however, and we greeted a few other people also walking on it.

This walk was obviously over an hour.

Trail Thirteen

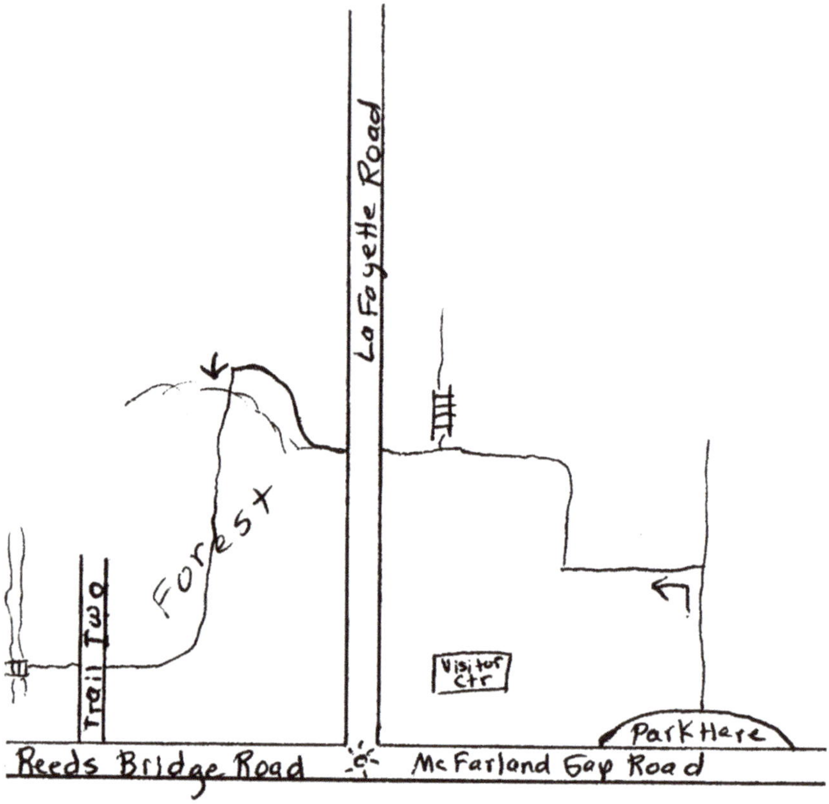

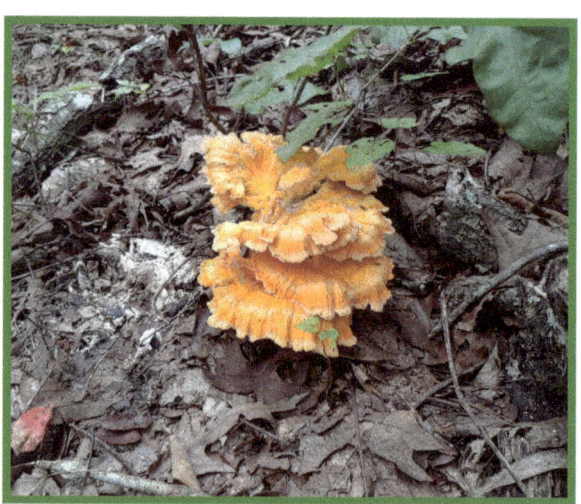

Fungi, lichen, and mosses make bright spots along the trails in all seasons.

TRAIL THIRTEEN
Hikers and people on horses will enjoy this trail, but it is too uneven for people in wheelchairs or with canes.

Location: Use the same entrance as described in TRAIL TWELVE. It starts about six minutes in, and is the left turn described in TRAIL TWELVE which made reference to this trail.

TRAIL THIRTEEN continues through the woods; watch your step in some places. It opens onto the field where you can see the Visitors' Center about a quarter of a mile away. It then narrows down to a narrow horse trail which follows the edge of the woods down to a trail which comes from a field parking lot to the Visitors' Center and crosses a wooden bridge. Some yards before the bridge is a hitching post where people can tie their horses and let them rest.

After TRAIL THIRTEEN crosses the trail with the yellowish wooden bridge, it then continues and goes under the LaFayette Road bridge. The small creek is fairly easy to cross. It then comes out on the other side of the road where the large Florida monument with the statue of a man under a shelter is.

A marker says horses, hikers, but no bikes. Further down the field is a large Illinois marker. As you become parallel with the Illinois marker, the horse trail continues down, but to the left is a trail marker going into the woods. The marker here says hikers or people with dogs, but no bikes or horses.

We took the trail going into the woods. About eight minutes later, we crossed over the hiker trail marker near Reeds Bridge Road described in TRAIL TWO, and continued straight until we reached a wooden bridge crossing the creek.

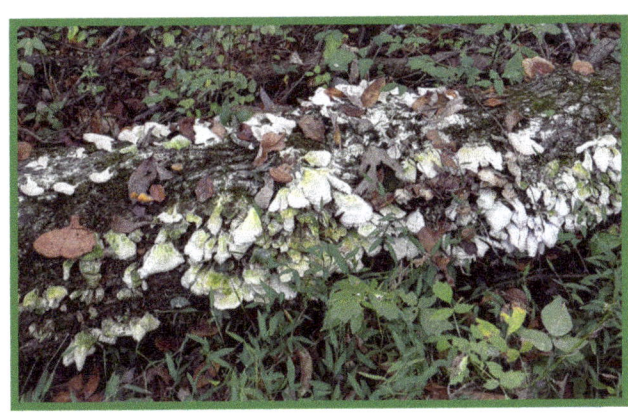

An estimate for TRAIL THIRTEEN to this point would be about forty-five minutes.

38 Accessible Trails in Chickamauga Park

Trail Fourteen

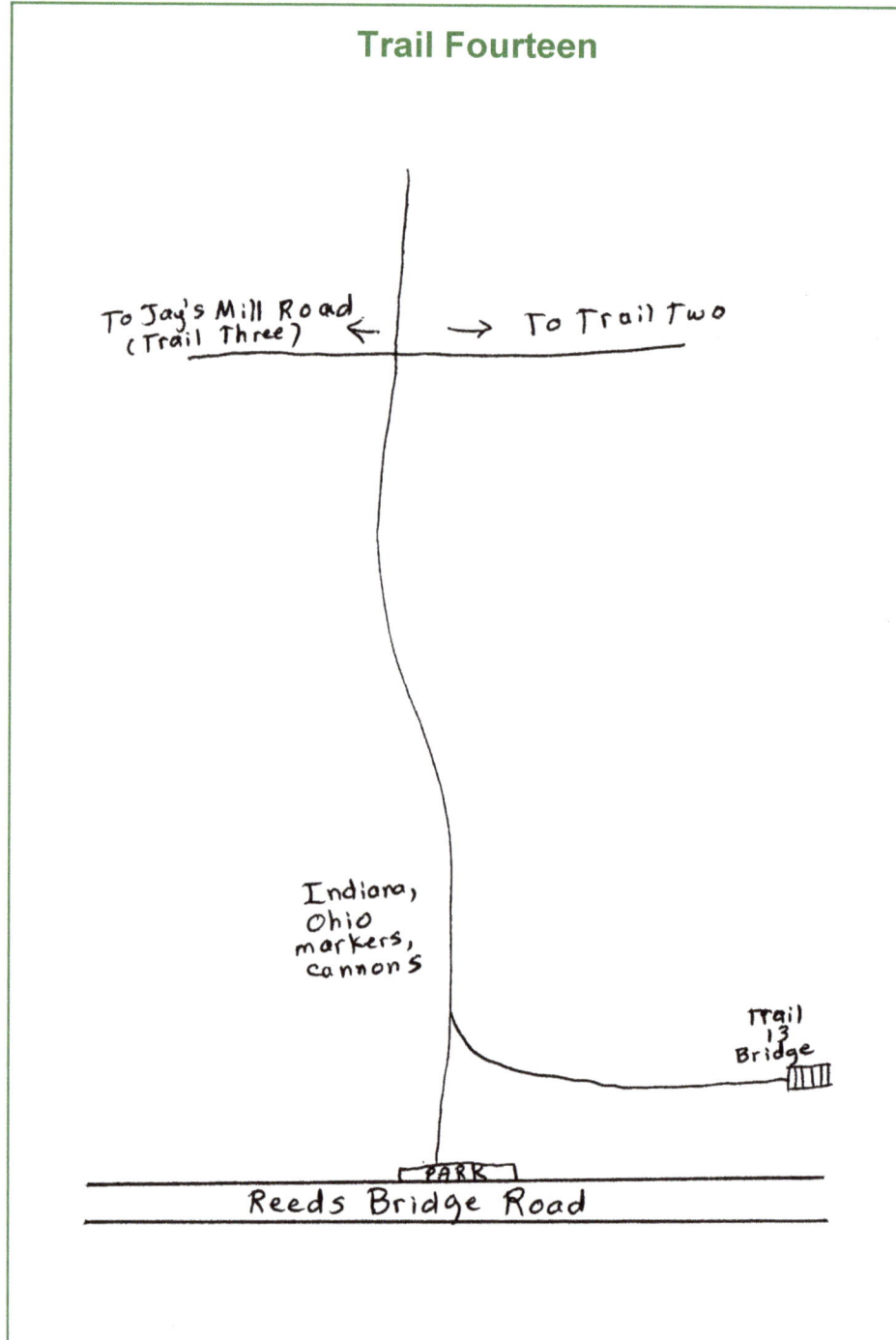

TRAIL FOURTEEN

The park sign at the entrance says horses, hikers, dogs on leash. No bikes. I don't recommend wheelchairs or canes. You might go in a little way, but not far.

Location: This starts on Reeds Bridge Road at a parking area with five parallel parking places. The sign nearest the trail is a Union sign entitled, "Brannan's Division Thomas' Corps. Brig. Gen. John M. Brannan".

About six minutes in, on the left, is a marker, Indiana 82nd regiment infantry. Further down the same left turn is a 35th regiment Ohio infantry marker. This is a nice wide trail, but there are tree roots. It finally dead-ends with an Indiana 87th regiment infantry marker.

Back on TRAIL FOURTEEN, on down also on left are two cannons with a blue marker, "USA – Church's Michigan Battery, 6 Guns. Connell's Brig. Brannan's Division…". Both of the cannons had rifling marks in them.

About 20 minutes into the trail, we came to an intersection. The left turn goes to Jay's Mill Road (TRAIL THREE.) Going straight is the left turn at the intersection mentioned in TRAIL THREE. Going right will eventually go to TRAIL TWO.

We turned around and went back past the six-minute turn with the Indiana and Ohio markers, and came to a V-shaped intersection.

The way back to the parking lot was marked for hikers and horses, but we went left on the trail marked "Hiker trail – Bikes and horses prohibited." This trail goes in a gradual descent, and you can see the traffic on Reeds Bridge Road through the trees. It finally comes to the bridge mentioned in TRAIL THIRTEEN. If we crossed this bridge and went on, we would eventually also come to TRAIL TWO.

40   Accessible Trails in Chickamauga Park

PROJECT CERTIFICATE

MY NAME _____

For purposes of safety, it is highly recommended to have a hiking partner on each trail.

Three goals are described below, Not everyone will have time for all fourteen trails or be able to complete them, so three curses are suggested below, or write in your own.

A   Reed's Bridge goal - complete five trails below
      Date completed _____

B.   Battle Line Road goal - complete ten trails below
      Date completed _____

C   Alexanders' Bridge Goal - complete all fourteen trails below
      Date completed _____

D   Other (describe) _____
      Date completed _____

TRAIL	DATE	MY HIKING PARTNER
TRAIL ONE	_____	_____
TRAIL TWO	_____	_____
TRAIL THREE	_____	_____
TRAIL FOUR	_____	_____
TRAIL FIVE	_____	_____
TRAIL SIX	_____	_____
TRAIL SEVEN	_____	_____

TRAIL   DATE   MY HIKING PARTNER

TRAIL EIGHT   _____   _____

TRAIL NINE   _____   _____

TRAIL TEN   _____   _____

TRAIL ELEVEN   _____   _____

TRAIL TWELVE   _____   _____

TRAIL THIRTEEN   _____   _____

TRAIL FOURTEEN   _____   _____

PROJECT CERTIFICATE

MY NAME _____

For purposes of safety, it is highly recommended to have a hiking partner on each trail.

Three goals are described below, Not everyone will have time for all fourteen trails or be able to complete them, so three curses are suggested below, or write in your own.

A   Reed's Bridge goal - complete five trails below
       Date completed _____

B.   Battle Line Road goal - complete ten trails below
       Date completed _____

C   Alexanders' Bridge Goal - complete all fourteen trails below
       Date completed _____

D   Other (describe) _____
       Date completed _____

TRAIL	DATE	MY HIKING PARTNER
TRAIL ONE	_____	_____
TRAIL TWO	_____	_____
TRAIL THREE	_____	_____
TRAIL FOUR	_____	_____
TRAIL FIVE	_____	_____
TRAIL SIX	_____	_____
TRAIL SEVEN	_____	_____

TRAIL	DATE	MY HIKING PARTNER
TRAIL EIGHT	_____	_____
TRAIL NINE	_____	_____
TRAIL TEN	_____	_____
TRAIL ELEVEN	_____	_____
TRAIL TWELVE	_____	_____
TRAIL THIRTEEN	_____	_____
TRAIL FOURTEEN	_____	_____

ADDITIONAL NOTES

ADDITIONAL NOTES

ADDITIONAL NOTES

www.ingramcontent.com/pod-product-compliance
Lightning Source LLC
LaVergne TN
LVHW010319070426
835512LV00023B/3479